MW01031841

Making Lotion:
The Heavy Winter Lotions

25 Lotion Recipe Guide for your Hobby or Business

A Thermal Mermaid Guide

By **Jennifer & Hannah Tynan**

Copyright 2016 © Jennifer Tynan

All rights are reserved. No part of this book may be reproduced in any manner whatsoever without written permission. Unauthorized reproduction of this work is illegal. No part of this book may be scanned, uploaded, or posted on the internet without the author's permission.

This book is not meant to take the place of medicine or medical advice from a professional. The contents in this book do not make guarantees in anyway and have not been reviewed or approved by the FDA like the commercial chemical products. As always nursing, pregnant women, and children should consult with your trusted doctor before consuming. There are always cautions and warnings about using essential oils when pregnant or nursing. Not all essential oils are suitable for babies and children.

The Lotion Recipe Collection from Thermal Mermaid is Broken Down into 3 Volumes

1. **Lotion Making: 25 Lotion Recipe Guide for Beginners Hobby or Business (Thermal Mermaid Lotion Book 1)**

This volume covers 25 recipes for lightweight summer time lotions

2. **Lotion Making: 25 Lotion Recipe Guide for Beginners Hobby or Business (Thermal Mermaid Lotion Book 2)**

This volume covers 25 recipes for heavy weight nourishing winter time lotions

3. **Lotion Making: 25 Lotion Recipe Guide for Beginners Hobby or Business (Thermal Mermaid Lotion Book 1)**

This volume covers 25 recipes for thick body butters and massage bars

Other Books in the Thermal Mermaid Collection

90 Soap & Bath Recipes: A Soap Making Guide for Hobby or Business (Book 1)

50 Spa & Treatment Products for your Home or Store (Book 2)

50 Cosmetic Products for Skin & Make Up: Cosmetics to Make for You or Your Store (Book 3)

Table of Contents

Introduction:

Welcome to part two of our lotion collection recipes. The lotion recipes made by Thermal Mermaid are broken into three parts. In this book, all of the recipes are going to produce a thicker heavy weight product. These lotions are often labeled night creams or firming creams. You can still pump them from a bottle, but they will not be runny and thin. These recipes are purchased more often in cold weather, and the recipes will lean more toward the holiday and winter months.

This short guide is meant for beginner to medium-advanced. If you are a follower of the Thermal Mermaid books you will know that the recipes in this book are our own and the ones we use when we take our crafts to our market tables. Every recipe is something that we have made and sold. We do constantly change and tweak our recipes and sometimes invent brand new ones. Also, we do not repeat recipes in our books. Many other of our books will also offer lotion recipes. We do try to offer creativity and variety, but they are always different from the recipes in our other books. We make recipes for those who want to make lotion at home, but also those who want to make products for a small business for their craft table or market. This means, look at the recipe amounts and do your reasoning accordingly. We may give a recipe for a small personal amount, or for a batch of 8 bottles. This is meant to be an example, and you will need to adjust as you see fit.

Safety First: In our full volumes we do go into greater detail about safety and protection, but we will repeat just a few points about safety and preparation of your products. Please forgive this if you are a loyal Thermal Mermaid reader, and understand that if this is the first book one had bought in our collection we feel that some things are important enough not to leave out for those who may just be starting.

Finally, you will see a few ingredients that you may not recognize if you are a beginner. Don't let this scare you away. Our recipes are for real lotions, not mock up lotion like products that you can make out of the kitchen in some DIY tutorial. Our recipes are products worth selling with your name on it. All of the ingredients are easily available in small amounts online, so you don't need to be a big brand and buy bulks of materials. You can buy some of these things in a small as 4 oz. quantities. Most of these funny names are just waxes that help blend the oils and waters together and keep things feeling smooth without your product falling apart.

What to expect in this Book?

This book offers 25 lotion recipes of just heavy evening wear or cold weather winter lotion. Each recipe is one that we have made, used, and sold at our market table.

We will also talk about our observations and pointers about some of these recipes. We will also tell you what you need to gather to make your products We will also offer you some pointers of where to get the best supplies online at the best costs.

Safety & Preparation

If you are a reader of Thermal Mermaid you will know that we do spend a good amount of time discussing our feelings about safety and preparing your products. Some forethought goes into making cosmetic before you even start. Unlike in soap making, you are not using lye, a caustic chemical, and you do not need the full break down on safety prevention. However, we do recommend that you use a preservative in your product, either Optiphen or Liquid Germall Plus.

Here are our pointers about preservatives.

First, these are chemicals that will make up no more than 2-5 percent of your recipe, but when you are handling it, you are handling it in its concentrated form so be a gem and wear gloves. It is a chemical.

Second, you may think to yourself, hmmm, I don't want to put a chemical in my products. The whole reason that people will buy from me instead of from the drug store is because my products are natural. You're probably correct. However, there are preservative that are harsher than others and there are some to steer clear away from. Those are parabens, SLS, and formaldehydes. The two we use are sold at your local soap supplier and do not contain these chemicals. Do not ever sell an item to a customer without a preservative. Lotions can grow mold if not made or stored correctly and you never want to risk someone rubbing bacteria into their skin, especially if their skin is broken, and you never know if someone's health is already compromised. Feel free to make any of these lotions for your own personal use without preservatives. Just know that they will expire like food and keeping your bottle in the fridge will make it last longer. When I make a small batch for myself I often do not use preservative. (Because it is expensive and I use it in my batches for sale. I have no qualms about using the preservatives that I sell on my own skin.) When I make my batch I never keep it for more than 2 weeks.

The final safety pointer is about your work space. Since you already know that lotions can breed bacteria, we must stress the sterilization of your jars, lids, and table tops. You need to spray down your packaging containers and utensils with a bottle of rubbing alcohol, then wipe away the moisture. You must wear gloves when making lotion. Remember, anything that you make where you introduce water into the ingredients can potentially breed bacteria. Lotions contain water so we need to keep a sterile environment. Never, never skip out on your cleaning duties when selling or gifting to other people.

One last note on packaging. Make sure your products are labeled correctly. In many places it is not permitted to sell items without a list of ingredients or labels. You need to do this if you plan to sell your things.

Items You Will Need

Bowls and Utensils – You will need a collection of bowls and whisks and spoons. You can expect that some recipes will call for mixing liquid, or dry materials, or setting one thing aside to cool while you work on something else. Just make sure you have a collection of bowls at hand.

Gloves – Don't ever make lotion without wearing gloves. This will reduce the risk of introducing bacteria to your product. It's a silly thing to not do correctly because a box of 100 gloves is sitting at your grocery store waiting for you for 5 dollars.

A spray bottle with rubbing alcohol – You need to spray and wipe your jars and lids. I completely trust you that your kitchen is well kept and sterile, but hey, it doesn't hurt to give your table top a once over.

Jars & Lids – You can use as many types of plastic jars and lids as you can find online to package. We recommend you buy this online because you will get the best prices. For the recipes in this book you don't really need the large mouth jars because the recipes are light and runny. You will either need pump bottles or squeeze bottles. One note: the containers and lids are often sold separately. Just pay attention when you are buying whether or not you have to put the matching lid to any jar in your shopping cart.

A stick blender – This will help emulsify your oils and waters together. It makes a big difference compared to a whisk.

Piping Bags – Plastic Piping bags that are meant for cake icing will be used to make some of the lotions with layered colors.

Clamps or Clothespins – I find these very useful for closing bags and products in a pinch. You will need these to pinch your piping bags when you are using them. (AH, if we only had 4 arms…)

Recipes

1. Nourishing Beeswax Hand Cream

What you will need:

- ½ cup Almond oil
- ½ cup coconut oil
- 7 oz. of shea butter
- .2 ounces of E-wax
- .5 ounces of bees wax
- .2 oz. of vitamin E oil
- .2 oz. of Optiphen
- 6 drops of Lavender Essential oil

Instructions & Notes: Beeswax is easy to get and often turns out to be that secret miracle ingredient when it comes to hardening your product. Lavender oil is a night time fragrance that sooths and aids in sleep.

This recipe will make two 8 oz. bottle, so adjust accordingly.

First, sanitize your environment, hands, bottles, and put on your gloves. Heat up your aloe juice in a pot. When you are working with small amounts, I find that this is easier to do in the microwave. You will need to melt your waxes into your oils. You can do this in short bursts in the microwave as well. It is easier to overheat in the microwave, so use good care just to give it enough heat to melt your ingredients.

Mix you aloe, waxes, and oils together with your stick blender. Allow plenty of time for that e-wax to bond the aloe and oils. You will find it is easier to keep the aloe juice together with the oils. It doesn't separate as readily as water does.

Allow this to cool. Then, add your fragrance and preservative. Mix well and pour into your bottles.

2. Goats Milk Lotion

What you will need:

- 2 oz. Steric Acid
- 2.4 oz. E-wax
- .4 oz. Sodium Lactate Preservative
- 1 tsp. Vitamin E
- 1 tbsp. of Glycerin
- 4 oz. of coconut oil
- 4 oz. of heavy green olive oil
- 18 oz. of pasteurized goats milk
- 18 oz. of distilled water

Instructions and Notes: Make sure all your working space is sterilized. Wear gloves. Boil and bleach your kitchen dishes and utensils if you can. Every item must be as sterile as possible. If your goats milk is fresh you will need to pasteurize it. You can do this you must bring it to a slow simmer at 164 degrees for 20 minutes. This will ensure to kill and bacteria in the goat's milk. If you are using the powdered goats milk, make sure you boil your distilled water before use.

In a large bowl, add the wax with all the oils and the shea butter. Stir together, and place in the microwave in short bursts. Take it out every 10 to 15 seconds and stir lightly. Repeat this until the wax has melted into the oil. This should be done slowly. Don't get the oils too hot, however the wax does require a little effort to melt.

In a cooking pot add the water and the goats milk. Pour the melted waxes and oils into the milk and water. Blend well with your stick blender. Continue for two or three minutes. You will notice that the lotion will start to become thick and creamy. Now it is time to add the preservative, glycerin, and vitamin E. Now is also the time to add a fragrance oil if you choose to add one. Return the stick blender and blend for an additional minute.

Once you have blended this you will fill the lotion bottles as soon as possible. This lotion is a thick recipe and will only become more thick as it cools further. Set a small kitchen funnel at the tops of your lotion bottle and pour 8 oz. of product into each one. This recipe will make 6 bottles of lotion.

Cap the bottles and wipe everything down before adding your labels. This lotion will be thick but still pliable to package in a squeeze bottle.

3. Almond Oil Lotion

What you will need:

- 30 oz. of water
- .5 oz. of preservative
- 1 oz. jojoba oil
- 1 oz. of argon oil
- 1 oz. of grapeseed oil
- .5 oz. of castor oil
- 8 oz. of almond oil
- 2 oz. of shea butter
- 4.5 oz. of E-wax
- .5 oz. of Optiphen

Instructions and Notes: This is a luxurious mid weight winter moisturizing lotion that is loved by my market customers. Do not fail to remember that there are people who have nut allergies, and even though we aren't making food, some people can't even come in contact with nut oils without an allergic reaction.

Therefore, keep this lotion labeled properly and don't forget to mention to your customers it contains nut oils when they buy from you in person. Sometimes people think that almond lotion means that it is just fragranced that way, but we are filling this recipe with actual nut oil.

Before we begin, sterilize your area, including the counter and your preparation utensils. Wear gloves, and boil your bottle lids. Spray down your lotion bottles with a spritz of alcohol solution. Kill all the potential germs.

Melt the wax and the shea butter in the microwave on short bursts. Mix all the oils in a bowl together. Add the melted e-wax and butter into the oil. Blend with your stick blender. Add the water and continue blending. You will start to notice the lotion becoming more thick. Add the Optiphen. Blend for 1 minutes. You can leave this lotion unscented if you want to, because the almond oil scent give this recipe a pleasant natural aroma.

Before the lotion sets, pour into 8 oz. bottles. Cap with the lids, and wipe the bottles down before placing the labels on the bottles. This recipe will make 6 - 8 oz. bottles of lotion.

4. Cherry Blossom Body Lotion

What you will need:

This body lotion is a thick lotion with a creamy butter consistency. It is a luxurious product that melts into your skin and moisturizes. This cherry blossom fragrance is a great break away from the seasonal holiday selections.

- 24 oz. of Water
- 5 oz. of Olive Oil
- 3.2 oz. of E-Wax
- 2.5 oz. of Evening Primrose Oil
- 2.5 oz. of Rose Hip Seed Oil
- 2.5 oz. of Steric Acid
- 1.5 oz. of Isopropyl Myristate
- .7 oz. of Optiphen Plus
- .5 oz. of Vitamin E
- .5 oz of Cherry Blossom Fragrance Oil
- 9 / 4 oz. jars with caps

Instructions and Notes: In a large bowl add the water, steric acid, and emulsifying wax. Melt these in the microwave until the waxes are completely melted. Only heat until the waxes are melted. Add the Olive Oil, Primrose Oil, and Rose Hip Seed Oil. Stir and allow the butter to softly melt. With either a hand mixer or stand mixer blend this mixture until it begins to thicken. Add the Vitamin E, Isopropyl Myristate and Cherry Blossom Fragrance Oil. Continue to blend for a few minutes. Next add your Optiphen Plus preservative. The temperature must be under 107 degrees so the preservative does not burn off before it is thoroughly mixed. Scoop the mixture into your jars. Allow your mixture to cool before capping so that you do not get condensed water drops inside the jars.

5. Heavy Hemp Lotion

Hemp oil has had some chatter for years now about its medicinal properties for several skin ailments. Hemp oil will leave skin feeling soft and smooth for hours. This is a soft, rich, heavy weight lotion recipe. When selling this type of lotion at your market table, there are two kinds of hemp shoppers. There are those who are interested in the holistic medicinal products of hemp seed oil, and there are those who are attracted to the "pot" novelty. Keep in mind when selling a "hemp" product, the average person isn't trying to smell like a novelty when they buy this. Try to steer away from making this lotion smell musky or heavy. Heavy weight lotions are for the colder seasons, lighter crisp scents make people feel clean and light under all those winter layers. Most people who are looking for hemp lotion are not looking for a product that is tinted green and smells like musk.

- 48 oz. of distilled water
- 5 oz. of Hemp Seed Butter blend
- 5 oz. of Hemp Seed Oil
- 3.2 oz. of E-wax
- 2.6 oz. of Steric Acid
- .5 oz. of Citrus Fragrance Oil

- .5 oz. of Crisp Linen Fragrance Oil
- .5 oz. of Vitamin E
- .66 oz. of Optiphen Plus
- 8 / 8 oz. clear bottles. With caps

Your work space must be properly sterilized and your bottles must be sprayed down with rubbing alcohol before adding your product. First, add your oils and butters to your water into your stand blender. Mix this well. Add your E-wax and steric Acid. Mix thoroughly, and add your remaining ingredients. Once these are blended well, fill your bottles.

6. Winter Shimmer Lotion

We love shimmer lotion. This will give you a touch of shimmer on your skin and add a brightened touch during the dull winter months. This is a popular item when matched with holiday theme products. The opal sparkle mica gives this product a frosty nutcracker theme

What You Will Need:

- 48 oz. of distilled water
- 6 oz. of Shea Butter
- 4 oz. of Olive Oil
- 3.2 oz. of E-wax
- 2.6 oz. of Steric Acid
- 1 oz. of Sugar Plum Fragrance Oil
- .5 oz. of Vitamin E
- .66 oz. of Optiphen Plus
- 8 / 8 oz. clear bottles. With caps
- 3 tsp of opal sparkle mica powder
- .5 tsp of powder blue mica

Your work space must be properly sterilized and your bottles must be sprayed down with rubbing alcohol before adding your product. First, add your oils and butters to your water into your stand blender. Mix this well. Add your E-wax and steric Acid. Mix thoroughly, and add your remaining ingredients. Once these are blended well, fill your bottles.

7. The Eczema Soothing Cream

This is a rich heavy lotion that will sink into the skin without leaving a greasy layer on the skin surface. Some people may need to apply lotion frequently in the winter months. This is wonderful for people who really need that deep medicinal lotion without feeling damp and sticky all day.

What You Will Need:

- 48 oz. of distilled water
- 4 oz. of Avocado Oil
- 6 oz. of Olive Oil
- 3.2 oz. of E-wax
- 2.6 oz. of Steric Acid
- 1 oz. of Love Spell Fragrance Oil
- .5 oz. of Vitamin E
- .66 oz. of Optiphen Plus
- 8 / 8 oz. clear bottles. With caps
- 3 tsp of opal sparkle mica powder
- .5 tsp of powder blue mica

Your work space must be properly sterilized and your bottles must be sprayed down with rubbing alcohol before adding your product. First, add your oils and butters to your water into your stand blender. Mix this well. Add your E-wax and steric Acid. Mix thoroughly, and add your remaining ingredients. Once these are blended well, fill your bottles. The Love Spell Fragrance is a dupe of the Victoria Secret brand. This is an extremely romantic floral fruity fragrance. Change the fragrance oil to a Woodland, or Sea Breeze to make this version for men.

8. French Vanilla After Shower Lotion

What You Need:

- 48 oz. of water
- 1 oz. of shea butter
- 1 oz. of cocoa butter
- 3 oz. of coconut oil
- 5 oz. of sunflower oil
- 2.5 oz. of steric acid
- 3.2 oz. of E-wax
- .5 oz. of Vitamin E
- .65 oz. of Optiphen preservative
- 20 ml of French Vanilla fragrance oil
- 10 ml. of Vanilla Color Stabilizer

Instructions and Notes: Prepare your sterile environment. In a large pot, add 48 oz. of distilled water. Bring the water to a slow boil over low heat. Measure the Stearic Acid and Emulsifying Wax and mix with the water. Allow this to melt slowly. Turn the heat off, and allow this to cool. Weigh out your oils and butters. While the water is still warm, add the butters and oils. Allow these to melt and mix with your stick blender. This will start to thicken as it cools. Next add Vanilla Stabilizer. Any fragrance with a vanilla fragrance has a tendency to turn your product brown, a stabilizer is recommended to keep your lotion its natural color. Add the Vitamin E and Vanilla Fragrance. Now, as the product cools you will add the preservative. Check the temperature of your product, it must be lower than 176 degrees before you add the Optiphen. Blend for one minute. Pour this product into your bottles as soon as possible. It is easiest to work with before it becomes too thick.

9. Men's Hand Lotion

What You Will Need:

- 24 oz. of Distilled Water
- 1 oz. of Argon Oil
- 2.3 oz. of Sunflower Oil
- 1 oz. of Cocoa Butter
- 1.6 oz. of E-Wax
- .65 oz. of steric acid
- .65 oz. of glycerin
- .2 oz of Vitamin E
- .32 oz. of Optiphen
- 1 oz. of coconut oil
- .5 oz. of avocado butter
- 1 oz. Sea Kelp and Agave Fragrance Oil

Instructions and Notes: Sterilize your surface, equipment, and bottles. Boil the distilled water to free it from any potential bacteria. In a microwave safe bowl add the butters and waxes. Melt this on short blasts. Add the oils to the water. Blend with the stick blender. Add the melted wax mixture. Blend well. This will begin to thicken as you

mix. Add the vitamin E, and Optiphen. Blend well. Add the fragrance oil. Blend again. Bottle this product before it becomes too thick. Use a funnel to pour into the product bottles.

10. Men's Hand Lotion

What You Will Need:

- 24 oz. of Distilled Water
- 1 oz. of Argon Oil
- 2.3 oz. of Sunflower Oil
- 1 oz. of Cocoa Butter
- 1.6 oz. of E-Wax
- .65 oz. of steric acid
- .65 oz. of glycerin
- .2 oz of Vitamin E
- .32 oz. of Optiphen
- 1 oz. of coconut oil
- .5 oz. of avocado butter
- 1 oz. Sea Kelp and Agave Fragrance Oil

Instructions and Notes: Sterilize your surface, equipment, and bottles. Boil the distilled water to free it from any potential bacteria. In a microwave safe bowl add the butters and waxes. Melt this on short blasts. Add the oils to the water. Blend with the stick blender. Add the melted wax mixture. Blend well. This will begin to thicken as you

mix. Add the vitamin E, and Optiphen. Blend well. Add the fragrance oil. Blend again. Bottle this product before it becomes too thick. Use a funnel to pour into the product bottles.

11. Men's Hand Lotion

What You Will Need:

- 24 oz. of Distilled Water
- 1 oz. of Argon Oil
- 2.3 oz. of Sunflower Oil
- 1 oz. of Cocoa Butter
- 1.6 oz. of E-Wax
- .65 oz. of steric acid
- .65 oz. of glycerin
- .2 oz of Vitamin E
- .32 oz. of Optiphen
- 1 oz. of coconut oil
- .5 oz. of avocado butter
- 1 oz. Sea Kelp and Agave Fragrance Oil

Instructions and Notes: Sterilize your surface, equipment, and bottles. Boil the distilled water to free it from any potential bacteria. In a microwave safe bowl add the butters and waxes. Melt this on short blasts. Add the oils to the water. Blend with the stick blender. Add the melted wax mixture. Blend well. This will begin to thicken as you

mix. Add the vitamin E, and Optiphen. Blend well. Add the fragrance oil. Blend again. Bottle this product before it becomes too thick. Use a funnel to pour into the product bottles.

12. Men's Hand Lotion

What You Will Need:

- 24 oz. of Distilled Water
- 1 oz. of Argon Oil
- 2.3 oz. of Sunflower Oil
- 1 oz. of Cocoa Butter
- 1.6 oz. of E-Wax
- .65 oz. of steric acid
- .65 oz. of glycerin
- .2 oz of Vitamin E
- .32 oz. of Optiphen
- 1 oz. of coconut oil
- .5 oz. of avocado butter
- 1 oz. Sea Kelp and Agave Fragrance Oil

Instructions and Notes: Sterilize your surface, equipment, and bottles. Boil the distilled water to free it from any potential bacteria. In a microwave safe bowl add the butters and waxes. Melt this on short blasts. Add the oils to the water. Blend with the stick blender. Add the melted wax mixture.

Blend well. This will begin to thicken as you mix. Add the vitamin E, and Optiphen. Blend well. Add the fragrance oil. Blend again. Bottle this product before it becomes too thick. Use a funnel to pour into the product bottles.

13. Men's Hand Lotion

What You Will Need:

- 24 oz. of Distilled Water
- 1 oz. of Argon Oil
- 2.3 oz. of Sunflower Oil
- 1 oz. of Cocoa Butter
- 1.6 oz. of E-Wax
- .65 oz. of steric acid
- .65 oz. of glycerin
- .2 oz of Vitamin E
- .32 oz. of Optiphen
- 1 oz. of coconut oil
- .5 oz. of avocado butter
- 1 oz. Sea Kelp and Agave Fragrance Oil

Instructions and Notes: Sterilize your surface, equipment, and bottles. Boil the distilled water to free it from any potential bacteria. In a microwave safe bowl add the butters and waxes. Melt this on short blasts. Add the oils to the water. Blend with the stick blender. Add the melted wax mixture.

Blend well. This will begin to thicken as you mix. Add the vitamin E, and Optiphen. Blend well. Add the fragrance oil. Blend again. Bottle this product before it becomes too thick. Use a funnel to pour into the product bottles.

14. Men's Hand Lotion

What You Will Need:

- 24 oz. of Distilled Water
- 1 oz. of Argon Oil
- 2.3 oz. of Sunflower Oil
- 1 oz. of Cocoa Butter
- 1.6 oz. of E-Wax
- .65 oz. of steric acid
- .65 oz. of glycerin
- .2 oz of Vitamin E
- .32 oz. of Optiphen
- 1 oz. of coconut oil
- .5 oz. of avocado butter
- 1 oz. Sea Kelp and Agave Fragrance Oil

Instructions and Notes: Sterilize your surface, equipment, and bottles. Boil the distilled water to free it from any potential bacteria. In a microwave safe bowl add the butters and waxes. Melt this on short blasts. Add the oils to the water. Blend with the stick blender. Add the melted wax mixture.

Blend well. This will begin to thicken as you mix. Add the vitamin E, and Optiphen. Blend well. Add the fragrance oil. Blend again. Bottle this product before it becomes too thick. Use a funnel to pour into the product bottles.

15. Men's Hand Lotion

What You Will Need:

- 24 oz. of Distilled Water
- 1 oz. of Argon Oil
- 2.3 oz. of Sunflower Oil
- 1 oz. of Cocoa Butter
- 1.6 oz. of E-Wax
- .65 oz. of steric acid
- .65 oz. of glycerin
- .2 oz of Vitamin E
- .32 oz. of Optiphen
- 1 oz. of coconut oil
- .5 oz. of avocado butter
- 1 oz. Sea Kelp and Agave Fragrance Oil

Instructions and Notes: Sterilize your surface, equipment, and bottles. Boil the distilled water to free it from any potential bacteria. In a microwave safe bowl add the butters and waxes. Melt this on short blasts. Add the oils to the water. Blend with the stick blender. Add the melted wax mixture.

Blend well. This will begin to thicken as you mix. Add the vitamin E, and Optiphen. Blend well. Add the fragrance oil. Blend again. Bottle this product before it becomes too thick. Use a funnel to pour into the product bottles.

16. Men's Hand Lotion

What You Will Need:

- 24 oz. of Distilled Water
- 1 oz. of Argon Oil
- 2.3 oz. of Sunflower Oil
- 1 oz. of Cocoa Butter
- 1.6 oz. of E-Wax
- .65 oz. of steric acid
- .65 oz. of glycerin
- .2 oz of Vitamin E
- .32 oz. of Optiphen
- 1 oz. of coconut oil
- .5 oz. of avocado butter
- 1 oz. Sea Kelp and Agave Fragrance Oil

Instructions and Notes: Sterilize your surface, equipment, and bottles. Boil the distilled water to free it from any potential bacteria. In a microwave safe bowl add the butters and waxes. Melt this on short blasts. Add the oils to the water. Blend with the stick blender. Add the melted wax mixture.

Blend well. This will begin to thicken as you mix. Add the vitamin E, and Optiphen. Blend well. Add the fragrance oil. Blend again. Bottle this product before it becomes too thick. Use a funnel to pour into the product bottles.

17. Men's Hand Lotion

What You Will Need:

- 24 oz. of Distilled Water
- 1 oz. of Argon Oil
- 2.3 oz. of Sunflower Oil
- 1 oz. of Cocoa Butter
- 1.6 oz. of E-Wax
- .65 oz. of steric acid
- .65 oz. of glycerin
- .2 oz of Vitamin E
- .32 oz. of Optiphen
- 1 oz. of coconut oil
- .5 oz. of avocado butter
- 1 oz. Sea Kelp and Agave Fragrance Oil

Instructions and Notes: Sterilize your surface, equipment, and bottles. Boil the distilled water to free it from any potential bacteria. In a microwave safe bowl add the butters and waxes. Melt this on short blasts. Add the oils to the water. Blend with the stick blender. Add the melted wax mixture.

Blend well. This will begin to thicken as you mix. Add the vitamin E, and Optiphen. Blend well. Add the fragrance oil. Blend again. Bottle this product before it becomes too thick. Use a funnel to pour into the product bottles.

18. Men's Hand Lotion

What You Will Need:

- 24 oz. of Distilled Water
- 1 oz. of Argon Oil
- 2.3 oz. of Sunflower Oil
- 1 oz. of Cocoa Butter
- 1.6 oz. of E-Wax
- .65 oz. of steric acid
- .65 oz. of glycerin
- .2 oz of Vitamin E
- .32 oz. of Optiphen
- 1 oz. of coconut oil
- .5 oz. of avocado butter
- 1 oz. Sea Kelp and Agave Fragrance Oil

Instructions and Notes: Sterilize your surface, equipment, and bottles. Boil the distilled water to free it from any potential bacteria. In a microwave safe bowl add the butters and waxes. Melt this on short blasts. Add the oils to the water. Blend with the stick blender. Add the melted wax mixture.

Blend well. This will begin to thicken as you mix. Add the vitamin E, and Optiphen. Blend well. Add the fragrance oil. Blend again. Bottle this product before it becomes too thick. Use a funnel to pour into the product bottles.

19. Men's Hand Lotion

What You Will Need:

- 24 oz. of Distilled Water
- 1 oz. of Argon Oil
- 2.3 oz. of Sunflower Oil
- 1 oz. of Cocoa Butter
- 1.6 oz. of E-Wax
- .65 oz. of steric acid
- .65 oz. of glycerin
- .2 oz of Vitamin E
- .32 oz. of Optiphen
- 1 oz. of coconut oil
- .5 oz. of avocado butter
- 1 oz. Sea Kelp and Agave Fragrance Oil

Instructions and Notes: Sterilize your surface, equipment, and bottles. Boil the distilled water to free it from any potential bacteria. In a microwave safe bowl add the butters and waxes. Melt this on short blasts. Add the oils to the water. Blend with the stick blender. Add the melted wax mixture.

Blend well. This will begin to thicken as you mix. Add the vitamin E, and Optiphen. Blend well. Add the fragrance oil. Blend again. Bottle this product before it becomes too thick. Use a funnel to pour into the product bottles.

20.Men's Hand Lotion

What You Will Need:

- 24 oz. of Distilled Water
- 1 oz. of Argon Oil
- 2.3 oz. of Sunflower Oil
- 1 oz. of Cocoa Butter
- 1.6 oz. of E-Wax
- .65 oz. of steric acid
- .65 oz. of glycerin
- .2 oz of Vitamin E
- .32 oz. of Optiphen
- 1 oz. of coconut oil
- .5 oz. of avocado butter
- 1 oz. Sea Kelp and Agave Fragrance Oil

Instructions and Notes: Sterilize your surface, equipment, and bottles. Boil the distilled water to free it from any potential bacteria. In a microwave safe bowl add the butters and waxes. Melt this on short blasts. Add the oils to the water. Blend with the stick blender. Add the melted wax mixture. Blend well. This will begin to thicken as you

mix. Add the vitamin E, and Optiphen. Blend well. Add the fragrance oil. Blend again. Bottle this product before it becomes too thick. Use a funnel to pour into the product bottles.

21. Men's Hand Lotion

What You Will Need:

- 24 oz. of Distilled Water

- 1 oz. of Argon Oil

- 2.3 oz. of Sunflower Oil

- 1 oz. of Cocoa Butter

- 1.6 oz. of E-Wax

- .65 oz. of steric acid

- .65 oz. of glycerin

- .2 oz of Vitamin E

- .32 oz. of Optiphen

- 1 oz. of coconut oil

- .5 oz. of avocado butter

- 1 oz. Sea Kelp and Agave Fragrance Oil

Instructions and Notes: Sterilize your surface, equipment, and bottles. Boil the distilled water to free it from any potential bacteria. In a microwave safe bowl add the butters and waxes. Melt this on short blasts. Add the oils to the water. Blend with the stick blender. Add the melted wax mixture.

Blend well. This will begin to thicken as you mix. Add the vitamin E, and Optiphen. Blend well. Add the fragrance oil. Blend again. Bottle this product before it becomes too thick. Use a funnel to pour into the product bottles.

22. Men's Hand Lotion

What You Will Need:

- 24 oz. of Distilled Water
- 1 oz. of Argon Oil
- 2.3 oz. of Sunflower Oil
- 1 oz. of Cocoa Butter
- 1.6 oz. of E-Wax
- .65 oz. of steric acid
- .65 oz. of glycerin
- .2 oz of Vitamin E
- .32 oz. of Optiphen
- 1 oz. of coconut oil
- .5 oz. of avocado butter
- 1 oz. Sea Kelp and Agave Fragrance Oil

Instructions and Notes: Sterilize your surface, equipment, and bottles. Boil the distilled water to free it from any potential bacteria. In a microwave safe bowl add the butters and waxes. Melt this on short blasts. Add the oils to the water. Blend with the stick blender. Add the melted wax mixture.

Blend well. This will begin to thicken as you mix. Add the vitamin E, and Optiphen. Blend well. Add the fragrance oil. Blend again. Bottle this product before it becomes too thick. Use a funnel to pour into the product bottles.

23. Men's Hand Lotion

What You Will Need:

- 24 oz. of Distilled Water
- 1 oz. of Argon Oil
- 2.3 oz. of Sunflower Oil
- 1 oz. of Cocoa Butter
- 1.6 oz. of E-Wax
- .65 oz. of steric acid
- .65 oz. of glycerin
- .2 oz of Vitamin E
- .32 oz. of Optiphen
- 1 oz. of coconut oil
- .5 oz. of avocado butter
- 1 oz. Sea Kelp and Agave Fragrance Oil

Instructions and Notes: Sterilize your surface, equipment, and bottles. Boil the distilled water to free it from any potential bacteria. In a microwave safe bowl add the butters and waxes. Melt this on short blasts. Add the oils to the water. Blend with the stick blender. Add the melted wax mixture.

Blend well. This will begin to thicken as you mix. Add the vitamin E, and Optiphen. Blend well. Add the fragrance oil. Blend again. Bottle this product before it becomes too thick. Use a funnel to pour into the product bottles.

24. Men's Hand Lotion

What You Will Need:

- 24 oz. of Distilled Water
- 1 oz. of Argon Oil
- 2.3 oz. of Sunflower Oil
- 1 oz. of Cocoa Butter
- 1.6 oz. of E-Wax
- .65 oz. of steric acid
- .65 oz. of glycerin
- .2 oz of Vitamin E
- .32 oz. of Optiphen
- 1 oz. of coconut oil
- .5 oz. of avocado butter
- 1 oz. Sea Kelp and Agave Fragrance Oil

Instructions and Notes: Sterilize your surface, equipment, and bottles. Boil the distilled water to free it from any potential bacteria. In a microwave safe bowl add the butters and waxes. Melt this on short blasts. Add the oils to the water. Blend with the stick blender. Add the melted wax mixture.

Blend well. This will begin to thicken as you mix. Add the vitamin E, and Optiphen. Blend well. Add the fragrance oil. Blend again. Bottle this product before it becomes too thick. Use a funnel to pour into the product bottles.

25. Men's Hand Lotion

What You Will Need:

- 24 oz. of Distilled Water

- 1 oz. of Argon Oil

- 2.3 oz. of Sunflower Oil

- 1 oz. of Cocoa Butter

- 1.6 oz. of E-Wax

- .65 oz. of steric acid

- .65 oz. of glycerin

- .2 oz of Vitamin E

- .32 oz. of Optiphen

- 1 oz. of coconut oil

- .5 oz. of avocado butter

- 1 oz. Sea Kelp and Agave Fragrance Oil

Instructions and Notes: Sterilize your surface, equipment, and bottles. Boil the distilled water to free it from any potential bacteria. In a microwave safe bowl add the butters and waxes. Melt this on short blasts. Add the oils to the water. Blend with the stick blender. Add the melted wax mixture.

Blend well. This will begin to thicken as you mix. Add the vitamin E, and Optiphen. Blend well. Add the fragrance oil. Blend again. Bottle this product before it becomes too thick. Use a funnel to pour into the product bottles.

Where to Get the Ingredients

Please remember, in full disclosure, my daughter and I own the store ThermalMermaid.com which makes soaps and cosmetics. We are not suppliers and we do not own these stores that we recommend. This is the list of suppliers I use and trust based on my experience. I am not related to any of these store owners and have never met them, so I can not 100% guarantee your experience but I am happy to share my resources and information with you.

TheSage.com – Majestic Mountain Sage – We buy dried flowers and herbs here. I have bought from other places online including overseas and the quality is always the best along with the price from this company. I have not bought anything other than dried roses, calendula, and chamomile flower buds, but I have watched many hours of videos from other craft makers online and I have only heard excellent recommendations from their products.

EssentialDepot.com – Essential Depot is a great place to get items such as Essential Oils, Fragrances, Oils, Butters, Molds. Essential Depot offers some of the most competitive prices and best shipping offers. This is the first website we shop at before any others. The quality of their product has never disappointed.

BulkApothecary.com – This website will provide you with mica, colorant, and jars with lids

About The Author

Jennifer Tynan grew up on the New England seaboard. She spent 10 years sub-contracting as an archeological field tech for environmental companies throughout the United States. She received a bachelor in Anthropology from the University of Connecticut.

With her daughter, Hannah, Jennifer spends some of her time making handmade artisan soap for her Bath and Body Company, Thermal Mermaid. Thermal Mermaid is an outdoor market found at summer vendors and renaissance fairs in New England. For those who are far away, products from Thermal Mermaid can be found on line. Many of the same recipes in this book are found on their product line.

Hannah is co-owner of Thermal Mermaid. At sixteen years old she is active in preparing and creating new product as well as organizing and developing her recipes. Hannah can often be found proudly sitting behind her market tables on the weekends while she studies her normal school work during the week. Hannah is a natural artist and is always working at designing creative packaging along with her soap recipes.

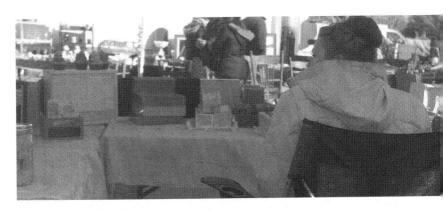

Hannah Sits behind her market display on a cold New England morning in early April.

Find us on Periscope and snapchat @ThermalMermaid where we go live and make our soaps and cosmetics for everyone. During this time, we can interact live.

Or Look us up on Facebook under Thermal Mermaid also

Sneak Peak

If you found the information in this book helpful, please explore a sneak peek at our first publication. This is a much longer book that goes into detail about safety and ingredients. You will find other lotion recipes in this book, but we do not repeat our recipes in the actual book itself.

90 Homemade Soap & Bath Recipes: Thermal Mermaid's Artisan Soap Makers Book

The Artisan Soap Makers Book is more than just a 'how to' on soap making for the beginner. It is a step by step introduction of creating an item that can be prepared, packaged, and sold for the purpose of building a small hobby business. The information in this book will provide hands on step by step instructions on how to make detergent free bath products at home, but the ultimate goal of this book is to provide the properly motivated type to have access to ideas that will allow them to run a small business with a low barrier to entry and provide a potential income so that one can be a little more self-sufficient tomorrow than they are today.

What you will find in this book:

1. A step by step guide on soaps and bath products made at a quality that one can sell in their community.
2. A description of the bare bones cheapest way to make the basics for the beginner.
3. Over 100 recipes that you can use and tweak to make your products
4. A breakdown of everything you will need to get started.
5. A dictionary and explanation of all the possible ingredients you can use and how to use them.
6. Where to sell your products and how to prepare yourself to run a business.

7. Thinking about your profit. How to price your items.

This guide has an additional workbook available where you can write down your recipe pages and calculate costs. See the paper back copy version of this book to get the attached workbook. It will save you time and help you see the big picture in your business when you can see your calculations on pages side by side.

How to Use this Book

Soap making has become an increasingly popular hobby in the last few years, and one will find many great books on the shelves with hundreds of homemade recipes. This book is meant for the beginner who is looking for an affordable start up business and finds soap making in their realm of interest, and will hold your hand with explanations on how to create a product and how to start a business from almost nothing.

This book is meant to be a resource to be kept for easy access, but it will also go one step further than an average soap "cookbook". This resource will show you how to break down and record your recipes so that you know exactly how much you are spending on each individual product you create so you know exactly how much you need to price each item at in order to run your business. This book is for the heart of the business man, not the at home mom looking for an afterschool activity with the kids. If you are the latter, simply go over to your local craft and hobby shop and find the one or two small shelves with melt and pour glycerin and plastic disposable molds and read the back of the package for instructions. You can make a few bars of soap with the kids for fun and be cleaned up in less than an hour. If you are interested in making this a small on the side business that could turn into something else, read on.

90 Homemade Soap & Bath Recipes: Thermal Mermaid's Artisan Soap Makers Book

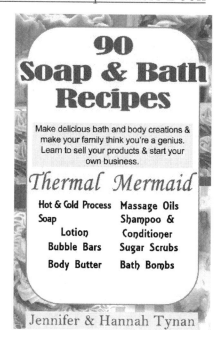

90
Soap & Bath
Recipes

Make delicious bath and body creations &
make your family think you're a genius.
Learn to sell your products & start your
own business.

Thermal Mermaid

Hot & Cold Process   Massage Oils
Soap   Shampoo &
    Lotion   Conditioner
Bubble Bars   Sugar Scrubs
Body Butter   Bath Bombs

Jennifer & Hannah Tynan

34640284R00044

Made in the USA
San Bernardino, CA
03 May 2019